# The Correctional Nurse Manifesto

## Other books by Lorry Schoenly

*Quick Start for Correctional Nurses:*
*Is Correctional Nursing for You?*

*The Wizard of Oz Guide*
*to Correctional Nursing*

*Correctional Health Care*
*Patient Safety Handbook*

*The Correctional Nurse Manifesto*

*Essentials of Correctional Nursing*

# The Correctional Nurse Manifesto

**Lorry Schoenly, PhD, RN, CCHP-RN**
Correctional Health Care Consultant

**Enchanted Mountain Press**

# Contents

# Introduction

Correctional nursing practice is full of landmines. We often walk a dangerous path through a jungle of tangled and conflicting values and norms. A map is always a help in foreign territory. Over the last few years, I have had the opportunity to consult with correctional nurses in a variety of settings as they struggle to provide much-needed care to a potentially violent and unsafe patient population. As correctional nurses we must, at times, advocate for patient health needs in an environment of differing priorities and shrinking resources. It is easy to get discouraged and disconnected from the professional nursing values that originally provided meaning to our nursing practice.

By reading this book you will be able to:

- Describe key threats to professional correctional nursing practice

- Identify ways to practice safe, effective, and compassionate nursing in the criminal justice system

- Outline methods to avoid becoming a jaded, cynical, and dissatisfied correctional nurse

A manifesto is a declaration of intention, motives and values of a group. It provides a true-north reading for group members to revisit during times of uncertainty. It makes visible the meaning of professional being and action. Affirmation statements can re-center us to those values of importance. With that in mind, I would like to suggest seven affirmations for a Correctional Nurse Manifesto.

# The Correctional Nurse Manifesto

As a correctional nurse, I will:

- Treat inmates with the dignity and respect deserving of any patient

- Work within my scope of practice at all times

- Not become cynical to the health requests of my patient population

- Hold myself and my peers to the professional boundaries of practice

- Continually guard my own and other's physical and mental safety

- Speak up when I see ill-treatment of my patient population

- Be a force for good in the community in which I work

# Manifesto Proposition 1: Treating Inmates like Patients

## Correctional nurses treat inmates with the dignity and respect deserving of any patient

*Henry was a strapping hulk of a man — previously part of a motorcycle gang — convicted of kidnapping, rape and murder. He is known to scream obscenities at the nursing staff when they make rounds in the ad seg unit where he is housed, due to many rules infractions in the medium security prison where you work. Now you see his name on your sick call list as you prepare for the morning round.*

Henry, and many inmates like him, is a part of the patient population that most correctional nurses encounter day-in and day-out. They are not easy to care for and often not easy to face. Henry has done despicable things in his life and he isn't improving during his stay at your facility. The security officers don't think much of Henry and treat him with contempt. It would be easy to do the same. Is Henry deserving of treatment with dignity and respect? Many would say 'No'!

Yet, nurses working in the criminal justice system are in the profession of caring and are bound by an ethical code that values every human being. The American Nurses Association (ANA) Code of Ethics for Nurses states:

*"The nurse, in all professional relationships, practices with compassion and respect for the inherent dignity, worth and uniqueness of every individual, unrestricted by consideration of social or economic status, personal attributes, or the nature of health problems."*

Henry is definitely a unique patient. He presents with a low social status and some undesirable personal attributes. How can a correctional nurse overcome repugnance to these characteristics of an inmate like Henry in order to treat him like a patient? Here are some tips for treating every inmate, even those like Henry, with the dignity and respect deserving of any patient.

## Focus on Who You Are, Not on Who They Are

It can be difficult to deliver good nursing care when you focus on the 'worthiness' of the patient. In fact, who the patient is is less important than who we are. As correctional nurses we have signed on to provide "…protection, promotion and optimization of health and abilities, prevention of illness and injury, alleviation of suffering through the diagnosis and treatment of human response, advocacy, and delivery of health care to individuals, families, communities and populations under the jurisdiction of the criminal justice system" (ANA definition of correctional nursing). Just as lady justice delivers her service blindfolded, those in our profession must do the same. It is the definition of who we are.

## Ramp Up Your Valuing

Being reminded of the values basis of our profession is another way to overcome negative emotions toward distasteful patients. The ANA Code of Ethics for Nurses provides a helpful foundation for valuing. In particular, the inherent nursing values of human dignity and worth of every individual is emphasized. Even the patient who has committed the most evil of acts, then, is deserving of the nursing care we have been trained and employed to provide.

## Don't Look Too Closely

The less you know about your patient's crimes, the better. Some information can't be avoided. If you work in a maximum security setting, you know your patients have likely done something violent; but, leave your curiosity at the gate when you come on shift. Consider your nurse-patient relationship as a human-to-human intervention. Nurses working in other settings rarely know the criminal history of their patients. Does that hinder their ability to provide professional nursing care? Doubtful. Seek a mental perspective in your care interactions that strips away any value judgments about your patient's history or past lifestyle.

## See the Big Picture

Within the microcosm of the individual nurse-patient interaction rests a larger picture of compassionate care. The modeling that nurses provide in respectful communication and concern for patient welfare contributes to the civility of the larger institution. By being who we are meant to be as nurses, we are instruments for change within the workplace culture. We can make a difference by stepping up and doing the hard work of caring for patients like Henry.

## Pause to Ponder

- How do you find the motivation to provide nursing care to difficult patients?
- Are you dealing with a difficult patient right now?
- What one thing will you do differently this week?

# Manifesto Proposition 2: Staying Within the Scope of Practice

## Correctional nurses work within their scope of practice at all times

Do any of these situations sound familiar?

- An RN in a small jail is asked by an officer to 'clear' one of the inmates for take-down into a restraint chair because he has been kicking at his cell door for two hours.

- An LPN/LVN is assigned to complete intake physical assessments because the RN who usually has that assignment is on maternity leave.

- A medication technician gives an inmate an antihypertensive from another patient's card because he can't find the inmate's supply in the medication cart during a busy pill line in a housing unit.

These are just a few examples where nurses (and others) can wander into territory beyond the scope of their licensure while working in corrections. Unlike traditional settings, jails and prisons can seem like the

Wild West where the law can be unclear and licenses can be on the line. Most nurses working in traditional settings have the protection of clearly defined boundaries of practice. A hospital, for example, is organized around the practice of health care and an organizational structure bounded by licensure. Nurses work within these boundaries and know what they can and cannot do based on policy, procedure and operating guidelines.

## Know Your Scope

In the correctional setting, however, nurses can work among those who are less familiar with the boundaries of licensure and have misconceptions about the knowledge and experience of the health care staff they work with. In a command and control environment things can get out of hand. In the first situation, the nurse is certainly able to determine if the inmate has a condition that should be taken into consideration in a forced restraint, such as a prosthetic hip, a serious heart condition or severe asthma. The nurse, however, is not in a position to medically approve the use of a restraint chair and must make this clear to the requesting officer. In addition, depending on the context, the nurse may have an obligation to request mental health intervention prior to use of force. This is a sensitive issue, especially in a jail setting.

## Ask Questions

Health care provision in a correctional setting can be under-funded and under-staffed. Managers struggle to provide required care with the staff available. This can lead to breaches in judgment about licensure boundaries. Differences between LPN/LVN and RN licensure can be blurred. This is particularly true with regard to assessment. Although experienced LPN/LVN's may have the skill to perform physical assessments, licensure may limit the legal ability to do so. Placing an LPN/LVN in a position to work beyond their licensure places them at high risk and may require clinical judgment beyond their training or experience. In the second situation, the LPN/LVN should question the assignment based on a knowledge of licensure requirement.

## Avoid Work-Arounds

Correctional facilities rarely have onsite dispensing pharmacies. Many rely on mail-order or fax-and-fill systems to obtain patient medications. The medication administration process is complicated by security issues and remote locations for delivery. Some systems allow trained but unlicensed technicians to deliver routine medications to the patient population. However, even licensed staff are tempted to create work-arounds when delivering a high volume of medications over a short period of time. One common work-around in medication administration is borrowing medication from one patient for administration to another. Although seemingly harmless, making choices like this is equivalent to pharmacy dispensing and beyond the scope of nursing or unlicensed staff. In the third example, the medication technician should either provide the missing medication from stock in the exact dosage ordered, or delay administration until the situation is cleared up upon return to the medical unit.

Correctional nurses care for patients in an environment that can be unfamiliar and unappreciative of the legal boundaries of licensure. We have a responsibility to fully understand our own scope of practice and practice safely within that scope at all times.

## Pause to Ponder

- Have you seen correctional nurses placed in situations beyond their scope of practice?
- What would you do in each of the situations described above?

# Manifesto Proposition 3: Avoiding Cynicism

## Correctional nurses do not become cynical to the health requests of their patients

*The night nurse was called to a housing unit because one of the inmates seemed to be seizing. When the nurse arrived, the patient was seen on the floor passed out. Her cellmate had called for help. The officers arrived to see the patient flailing about and babbling before passing out.*

Correctional nurses have a particular struggle to remain objective in practice. Our patient population and care environment can lead us to become jaded and cynical. New nurses soon learn that some inmates seek services for reasons other than health needs. The prison culture can value manipulation, deception and secondary gain. Nurses can unwittingly get caught up in a 'game' inmates are playing. Once burned in such a situation, a nurse can assume all inmates are looking for an angle when seeking health care.

Yet, many a correctional nurse has also been burned by assuming a patient is 'faking it' or being deceptive only to find that their health need was very real. What can correctional nurses do to protect themselves from manipulation while also guarding against jaded cynicism?

# Reasons to be Skeptical

There are several reasons why cynicism so easily develops when dealing with our patient population.

- **Manipulation is a way of life.** By the time many of our patients arrive in the facility, they have lived a life based on distrust, manipulation and deception. It is how they view the world and how they have used their skills to obtain what they want.

- **Care may not be given if the symptoms are not severe.** Some of our patients don't think they will get the attention of officers or health care staff unless they exaggerate their symptoms. There may be a basis for their health care request but it may not be as severe as described or presented.

- **Health care is a way out of the facility.** Other patients see health care as an opportunity to travel to the free world for hospital visits or specialty appointments. Every outside visit has the potential for contact with family and friends, or even an opportunity for escape.

- **Special treatment can bring status.** In the stripped-down prison society, health passes for lower bunks, special shoes or lighter work details can bring status. Special food, like evening snacks for diabetics, or desirable medications, can be used for trade or barter on the prison black market.

- **Special treatment can bring safety.** Many inmates feel vulnerable and unsafe in general housing units. A medical or mental health diagnosis may bring a more secure housing assignment and greater safety.

# Ways to Remain Objectively Caring

Nurses working in correctional settings must understand the very real potential of deception in the patient population while maintaining a professional perspective on the nurse-patient relationship and the need to deliver appropriate health care. Here are several ways to remain objective when dealing with inmate-patient requests.

- **Listen to the patient.** Keep an open mind when listening to your patient. Truly hear what they are saying about their symptoms. Listen for full descriptions. Be sure to objectively document these symptom descriptions and the circumstances of their emergence. This documentation has at least two uses. First, it validates the actions you will take during this encounter. Second, it provides a history for use with ongoing encounters. If a patient is 'working the system', it can become clear over time with solid documentation of symptoms. Good communication among the health care team is important. Listening to the patient also validates concern to the patient. This may encourage accurate description of the symptom if exaggeration is an issue. Listening can help determine if safety is a concern.

- **Observe and document.** Good observation and assessment skills are required in corrections. Document all observations with a keen eye toward those that validate or invalidate the patient's stated symptoms. Accurate and thorough observations can help the healthcare team 'get to the bottom' of the symptoms, whether actual or fabricated.

- **Seek corroborating evidence.** Validation of symptoms can also be obtained from others. Officers may observe patient activities in the housing unit and the exercise yard. Other team members such as social services, psychology, or medical staff may have corroborating evidence. This is why an integrated medical record can be so important. Be careful, however, to limit observations to objective data. Opinions and attitudes about motivations such as 'drug seeking' or 'malingering' have no place in the medical record.

- **Do not make assumptions**. Even a patient who has invented illness in the past may have a serious medical need in a future encounter. It is unwise to assume that a patient is contriving the current symptoms. Every nurse-patient encounter deserves an objective evaluation.

## Why Avoid Cynicism?

Wouldn't it be easier to just assume patients are being manipulative and deceptive when they seek out healthcare? Some nurses think so. However, we forfeit our professional nursing values when we see every patient in this light. We are also risking missing important medical conditions and delivering substandard care that would be indefensible should a legal claim be brought. It is in our own best professional interests and in the best interests of our patients to develop skills in remaining both realistic about the characteristics of our patient population while remaining objective in our delivery of nursing care.

## Pause to Ponder

- Have you struggled with cynicism in your correctional nursing practice?

- How did you pull out of it? What will you do differently the next time you suspect a patient is 'faking it'?

# Manifesto Proposition 4: Maintaining Professional Boundaries

## Correctional nurses hold themselves and their peers to the professional boundaries of practice

I live in a rural community of dairy farms. In fact, on every side of our property and across the road are cattle pastures. They all have fences around the boundaries of each field. Mostly, the cows are pleasant and stay within their territory. Once in a while, however, a fence falls into disrepair and Bessie wanders out into our yard. What trouble that can cause! These placid animals may not be violent, but they can plod through flower beds, randomly plop 'fertilizer' where it isn't needed, and chew up the shrubbery.

The idiom that 'good fences make good neighbors' can also be applied to our nursing practice. Good fences make good nurses – especially in corrections. Setting boundaries in your interactions with patients protects both you and the inmates in your care.

Lorry Schoenly

# Why Good Nurses (Like Good Neighbors) Need Fences

Professional boundaries separate therapeutic behavior in a nurse-patient relationship from other behaviors which may be well-intentioned but are not therapeutic or part of professional nursing practice. The National Council of State Boards of Nursing provides a helpful graphic of a continuum of relationship with boundaries for nursing practice. Correctional nurses must find ways to remain within the bounds of the Zone of Helpfulness in order to remain safe and provide appropriate nursing care. Out-of-bounds relationship could include under-involvement or over-involvement in the relationship.

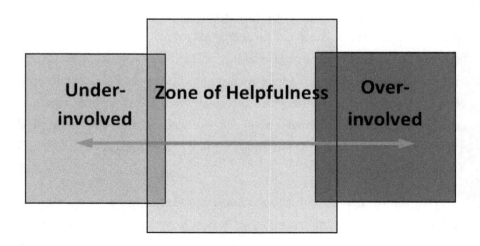

Correctional nurses can find themselves, or their peers, under-involved in patient relationships when cynicism or a jaded attitude to the inmate population takes hold. Under-involvement was discussed in Manifesto Proposition Three. Boundary blurring in correctional nursing practice can also lead to over-involvement in a patient relationship - moving toward a personal relationship that goes beyond the therapeutic role. Establishing a personal relationship with a patient is inappropriate, at best. It can be dangerous and illegal as well.

The Association of Registered Nurses of Alberta Canada published a helpful guide for the nurse-patient relationship that lists indications of boundary-crossing.

- Frequently thinking of the patient while away from work.

- Planning your day around the care of the patient.

- Sharing personal information or work concerns with the patient.

- Favoring the patient's care at the expense of others.

- Keeping secrets with the patient.

- Selectively reporting the client's behaviors (negative or positive).

- Changing dress style for work when working with the patient.

- Acting or feeling possessive about the patient.

- Swapping assignments in order to be with the patient.

- Feeling responsible for the patient if progress is limited.

These are the signs to look for in your own nurse-patient relationships and those of your peers. Make a pact with those you work with to call each other out if you see this behavior. Support each other in maintaining good fences in your correctional nursing practice.

Lorry Schoenly

# Broken Fences – Boundary Violations

Unfortunately, I see it again and again - correctional nurses crossing the boundary into sexual relationships, providing contraband, or drugs to inmate-patients. How does it happen? Boundaries are violated when a professional relationship moves to a social relationship. In a professional relationship, the nurse provides care and service based on using expert knowledge. The relationship is therapeutic and focused on the needs of the patient. A social relationship shifts this focus to personal needs and desires, thus distorting goals and intentions of communication and actions. At a minimum, this can be confusing to the patient and undermine therapeutic efforts. At worst, this can be exploitative and personally dangerous.

Boundary crossings lead to boundary violations. The line between a boundary crossing and a boundary violation can be blurred. Boundary crossings are single events in a nurse-patient relationship that may occur by error or lack of awareness. A boundary violation, however, is a persistent relationship characterized by indulging in actions of a personal nature. In the correctional setting, this often involves affectionate communication – both verbal and written (love letters); sexual interaction – touch, oral sex, intercourse; or providing contraband – drugs, cell phones, alcohol.

# Identifying Inappropriate Professional Behavior

We serve ourselves, our colleagues, and our patients by being alert for and responding to any indication of professional boundary crossing or violation. The College of Registered Nurses of Nova Scotia provides a decision-making framework with five quick questions to ask to determine if a behavior you are considering, or one you observe in a colleague, is within professional nursing boundaries. I have modified these questions to reflect American correctional nursing practice:

- Is the behavior consistent with the Nursing Code of Ethics?

- Is the behavior consistent with the Correctional Nursing Scope and Standards of Practice?

- Is the behavior consistent with your duty to always act in the best interest of your patient?

- Does the behavior promote patient autonomy and self-determination?

- Is this a behavior you would want other people to know you have engaged in with a patient?

If the answer to any of these questions is 'No' – DON'T DO IT!!!

## Mending Fences

Even if there have not been any boundary crossings or violations, good fence mending is in order. We all need to keep our professional fences in good repair and encourage our peers to do the same. Here are some recommendations from a recent nursing journal article on the subject.

- Openly discuss the challenge of professional boundaries with correctional nursing peers.

- Make a pact with your peers to 'watch their back' when it comes to observed boundary crossing. Look out for each other.

- Be particularly sensitive to stressful seasons in your personal life as this increases vulnerability to boundary violations in practice.

- Do not discuss intimate or personal issues with a patient.

- Do not keep secrets for, or with, patients.

- Treat all patients with dignity and respect (See Manifesto Proposition One).

- Speak, act and dress professionally to inspire professional conduct in yourself and others.

- Be firm, fair and consistent with all patients.

- Do not engage in behavior that can be misinterpreted as flirting – touch, personal compliments, etc.

## Pause to Ponder

- Have you seen indications of professional boundary violations in your correctional nursing practice or the practice of your peers?

- What will you do the next time?

# Manifesto Proposition 5: Physical and Mental Safety

## Correctional nurses continually guard their own and other's physical and mental safety

While professional boundaries can help protect a nurse's safety, correctional nurses must also be vigilant to guard against physical and psychological injury from a variety of sources on a daily basis. Officer, civilian and healthcare staff must provide a consistent front to protect against injury when dealing with the inmate population.

## Physical Safety

Workplace violence concerns are ever-present in the correctional setting. Correctional nurses need to be vigilant for physical injury from inmates, other staff or visitors. Here are some areas of concern for nurses:

- Know your facility's particular security procedures. This might include knowing security codes and procedures for obtaining assistance.

- Visually scan a work area or travel route for signs of safety threat. Avoid secluded areas or 'blind spots' within the facility.

- Travel in pairs or groups when possible. If you must travel alone, be sure that other staff members know your whereabouts and expected return.

- If you must travel alone, be within sight or sound of an officer at all times when in any inmate area. Know where the next officer station is on your route. Check in by a wave or 'Hello' with each officer to be sure they know you are traveling in the area.

- Dress conservatively to avoid misinterpretation. Choose loose-fitting, functional clothing and eliminate jewelry such as necklaces that can be a choking threat.

- Arrange exam rooms so that you are closest to the door to prevent entrapment.

- Be careful to keep confidential any security procedures such as pending shack-downs or cell searches.

- Keep close control of keys to secure areas. Lost keys can result in access to secure areas and physical threats.

- Do not discuss personal information around patients. Information about family members, schedules or personal stresses can be used for manipulation.

## Mental Safety

Many of our patients have developed patterns of subtle manipulation to gain control in relationships. These skills mean survival in the criminal world and can become a habitual mode of communication – even with healthcare staff. There are common themes to the manipulation patterns of inmate-patients. Be on guard for these manipulation techniques that come from the excellent book – The Art of the Con.

- **Staff Friendship.** Comments are personalized to establish a special relationship. "I am so glad you are here today. You are the only one who cares."

- **Peer Group Alienation.** Establishing a 'we vs. them' situation. "The night nurse is always complaining about you but I stuck up for you."

- **Request for Help.** A request for sympathy or an action beyond your nursing role. "Could you mail this letter to my 5-year-old son for me?"

- **Nudging.** A test to see how far you are willing to go beyond the rules. "Could I have a few alcohol wipes to clean my shaving equipment?"

- **Turnout.** Leverages past rules-breaking to request more serious offenses. "If you don't get me a cell phone, I'll have to report that letter you mailed for me last week."

## Looking Out for Others

Teamwork is a major part of delivering health care. It is also a necessary part of remaining safe in the correctional setting. We all need to be alert for our own safety, but also for the physical and mental safety of our workmates. It is usually easier to engage a peer in physical safety concerns, such as a reminder to keep the keys on their person or refrain from discussing personal information in a public area. However, it can be difficult to speak up when a fellow staff member is dressing provocatively or engaging in personal conversation with patients. Courage is needed. Your interventions in these areas, though, improve safety for everyone.

## Pause to Ponder

- Have you had to come to the aid of another staff member to protect them from physical or mental harm?

- Consider your last few inmate interactions. Can you see any safety concerns?

# Manifesto Proposition 6: Responding to Degrading Treatment

## Correctional nurses speak up when they see degrading treatment of their patient population

Nurses working in jails and prisons can be witness to brutality and indecencies in the course of providing health care. The nature of the correctional environment and the natural adversarial roles of inmates and correctional staff can lead to a pervasive culture of disrespect and indignity which is foreign to professional nursing practice. Over time, nurses can develop feelings of frustration, isolation and disempowerment. Or, even worse, correctional nurses can be socialized toward a negative orientation rather than maintain a professional nursing orientation. Survival in a harsh environment can involve desensitization to harsh and impersonal treatment or even a culture of cruelty. Recent news stories highlight the result of nurses who have identified with, and become socialized to, a dysfunctional culture to the detriment of their patients and their own professional practice.

# Crimes against Patients

In a Florida jail, nurses disregarded the pain and numbness complaints of a young male, resulting in permanent paralysis from a staph infection. In another case, a man suffering a stroke was left unattended for over a day in his cell before being transported to the local hospital and later dying. A third example involves the death of a man in a restraint chair after excessive pepper spraying. It is likely that nursing staff had contact with each of these patients. Were they privy to, or even a part of, the inflicted cruelty?

Nurses are called to make the health needs of their patients central. Our professional code requires compassionate and respectful treatment of all patients without consideration of social standing or personal attributes. The *Code of Ethics for Nurses* also calls us to promote, advocate for and strive to protect the health, safety and rights of our patients. How can we accomplish this in the correctional setting? We must speak up when we see ill-treatment of our patient population in the course of our work in the correctional setting.

# Silence is Not Golden

Avoiding conflict is common in the nursing profession. We are easily intimidated by those in power, whether they are the physician we take patient care orders from or the custody officer in charge of a housing unit. We may be working in an unhealthy or even hostile work environment due to conflicting values among the various disciplines.

Yet, silence is deadly, as we can see from the few examples above. In landmark work on the need to speak up in the traditional setting, less than

5% of surveyed staff was willing to confront a team member about abuse, disrespect, poor teamwork or incompetence. How can we garner the courage to speak out when we see degrading treatment of our patients?

## The Courage to Speak

Moral courage is the willingness to stand up for, and act according to, our professional values when they are being threatened. It is a skill that can be developed through intentional practice. Moral courage is necessary for successful correctional nursing practice. Often we are working in environments with a history of tolerance and indifference to the degrading treatment of others. Speaking up in the face of this work culture can be terrifying.

The following actions can help gather the courage needed to speak out against wrong treatment:

- Develop relationships within your work setting that allow you to speak up about how you are feeling about a difficult situation. It will be much easier to be heard in a critical situation if you have already developed a voice.

- Start small to develop your courage muscle. Speak up about small situations to practice for big ones. For example, mention rude behavior or harsh words immediately.

- Deal with the individual directly, and privately, before moving to engage management. Keep things local, when possible.

- If possible, have a suggestion for an alternative action to replace the ill-treatment. In the restraint chair/pepper spray situation above, a mental health consult may have been recommended.

- Know the proper process for reporting unethical treatment before it happens. How do you activate the chain of command on your shift? Who do you call or what is your first step?

- Talk about important nursing values with like-minded colleagues. Be allies in supporting each other to 'do the right thing' in the face of a moral issue.

## A Culture of Speaking

Correctional nurses have an opportunity to encourage an ethical culture by intervening when degrading treatment is witnessed. Each of us can be an instrument for good in the position we have within an organization. A single action can change a situation; can even save a life. We know this in the physiologic work we do every day. It is also true for the moral actions we take.

Are there correctional nurses working in the three facilities described above who wish they had responded or spoken up about the ill-treatment they witnessed? We may never know. As a correctional nurse, you may be placed in a position requiring moral courage to respond. Will you be ready?

## Pause to Ponder

- Have you seen degrading treatment of an inmate in your correctional nursing practice?

- Were you happy with your response? Would you do anything differently?

# Manifesto Proposition 7: Do Good

## Correctional nurses are a force for good in the community in which they work

*Heather works in a small jail where her Health Services Administrator and Medical Director are at odds. In addition, the deputies treat the inmates in a callous nature and security procedures are lax. Heather wants to do a good job for her patients and sees a lot of areas that could be improved with some attention. For one thing, new intakes with a known history of alcohol abuse are not being monitored closely. She is frustrated and feels like escaping back to the emergency room job she left a year ago.*

### It Just Takes One

*Never believe that a few caring people can't change the world. For, indeed, that's all who ever have.*

*Margaret Mead*

Correctional nurses can find themselves working in difficult environments for delivering good care. Competing priorities and friction among various disciplines can lead to great frustration. Barriers to delivering health care in a secure setting can make even simple nursing tasks into all-day efforts. Correctional cultures can emerge that lack good-will among staff and inmates alike. It can be hard to imagine that you, one nurse, can make a difference in a situation like Heather's. Yet, you never know what chain of events you set in motion by taking action in a situation. I am a firm believer that we are in every situation in our lives for a reason; known or unknown to ourselves. If we have concern over an issue, it is an indication that we should act on it for the good of all; by this we fulfill our professional roles and our ethical/moral human roles in the world.

## People Wait For a Leader

*We can choose to be affected by the world or we can choose to affect the world*

*Heidi Wills*

Group Mentality (or Herd Mentality) can cause people to be swayed into thinking and acting like the majority of their social circle. In the correctional setting, nurses can absorb the nature and mindset of the prevailing culture rather than maintaining their professional perspective. This can lead to lack of action in the face of inappropriate, harmful and even illegal activity.

Malcolm Gladwell in his highly recommended book, *The Tipping Point,* suggests that people don't act in the face of need in a group setting for two reasons. One reason is that they see that others are also experiencing this need and no one sees it as an issue. They conclude that they are misinterpreting what is happening. An example might be hearing an inmate crying out in pain and seeing no one else in the housing unit, including three officers, pay attention to it. A nurse might conclude that what she is hearing is not what she imagined.

Gladwell's second reason for individuals not acting when they come upon an individual in need in a group situation is because they assume that someone else must be taking care of it. He suggests that the responsibility to act is diffused among the group and no one feels a great enough need to act, assuming someone else in authority is probably taking care of it. In a group, people often wait for an indication from others as to how they should act. Be the person who does the right thing.

## Start Where You Are

*It is the greatest of all mistakes to do nothing because you can only do little - do what you can*

*Sydney Smith*

Correctional nurses are rarely in power positions, yet we have the power to take action that can lead to powerful good. Small actions can have big consequences. In the complex social structure of a correctional community, a courageous nurse doing the right thing can have a huge impact. Chaos Theory suggests that very small changes, such as the movement of a butterfly's wings, can change the course of our climate. We already know what the actions we take in our nursing practice, such as initiating an asthma treatment or identifying alcohol withdrawal, can do for our patients. Correctional nurses have the power to be a force for good in whatever environment we find ourselves.

## Pause to Ponder

- Have you had opportunity to be a force for good in a correctional setting?
- What one thing could you do today to make a difference?

# Taking on the Challenge

## "Knowing is not enough; we must apply. Willing is not enough; we must do" – Goethe

Correctional nursing can be the most difficult job you ever loved. When equipped with the right knowledge, skills and attitude you can make a difference in the lives of those who are marginalized and vulnerable. Many of us entered nursing to help people in need. I don't know of a needier patient population than those found in jails and prisons. Yes, some incarcerated patients can be difficult, unlovely and unlovable. Yet, each one is vested with the human dignity that requires nursing attention and care toward restoring health and well-being.

Will you sign on to the Correctional Nurse Manifesto? If so, please drop me a note at lorry@correctionalnurse.net and I will respond with a Manifesto Poster for your medical unit and subscription to my monthly newsletter.

# About the Author

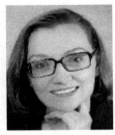 **Lorry Schoenly, PhD, RN, CCHP-RN**, is a nurse author and educator specializing in the field of correctional health care. She provides consulting services to jails and prisons across the country on projects to improve professional nursing practice and patient safety. She began her corrections experience in the New Jersey Prison System where she created and implemented education for nurses, physicians, dentists, and site managers. Before "accidentally" finding correctional healthcare, she practiced in critical care and orthopaedic specialties.

Dr. Schoenly actively promotes correctional nursing through social media outlets and increases the visibility of the specialty through her popular blog – correctionalnurse.net. Her podcast, Correctional Nursing Today, reviews correctional healthcare news and interviews correctional health care leaders. She is the recipient of the "B. Jaye Anno Award of Excellence in Communication" from the National Commission on Correctional Health Care.

CPSIA information can be obtained
at www.ICGtesting.com
Printed in the USA
LVHW021030231218
601529LV00020B/1060/P